"THANK GOD I ONLY HAVE TWO OF THESE!"

A collection of patients' writings gathered by a mammographer.

Susan E. Ghiassi R.T. (R)(M)(CT) (ARRT)

1

Dedicated to Zari, Gwen, women, and their families and friends everywhere.

ACKNOWLEDGEMENTS

First of all, a big thank you to my mammogram patients, past, present and future, who made this book possible!

A lot of love and thanks to my mom, June Miller, who at almost 86 years old drew the stick figures, edited and encouraged this book, and totally enjoyed reading the women's writings. And to her beloved husband, my dad, Boris Miller, who always thought I should write something. I love and miss them both.

Thank you to all my family, friends, co-workers at Raleigh Radiology Cedarhurst and Duke Raleigh Hospital Outpatient Imaging Center, neighbors, radiologists, and patients that helped me along the way to get this book ready for publishing: my brother and sister-in-law, Fred and Beverly Miller, my sister, Wendy Manion; my brother and sister-in-law, Andy Miller and Irene Eisenberg; Marina Pluta, Valencia High; the wonderful radiologists I work with at Raleigh Radiology Cedarhurst: Dr John G. Alley, Dr. Jennifer S. Van Vickle, Dr W. Kent Davis, Dr. Julia K. Taber; special friends that had a hand in this, too: Mrs. Judy Maschan, Ruth Donaldson, Krista Miller, Janice Whitley, Maryam Mahoutchian, Ruth Peterkin, Andee Baur, Sandy Marsh, Becky Ballard, Debbie Haefner, Maryam Davani, Tricia Parish, Soodi Ahmadi, Amanda Jorgenson, Moujan Khorram, Sharon DeSandro, Dana Davies, Elizabeth Gomez, , Mrs. Marj Wessen, Penny White, Alexis Eaves, Lynn Ruark,

Sandy Brainard, Dianne Baggett, Joanne Clayton, Julie McQueen, just to name a few. I know I pulled on many an ear, so forgive me if I've left you out.

June Kurtz, mammographer/friend, adjusted her schedule so I sometimes could take Zari to chemo treatments, I am so grateful to June.

Karen Hyman, dear friend, and my very first editor, who was encouraging from the beginning.

Arlene Summers, my neighbor/friend, who used her editing skills, listened, and said she could see this book happen!

Richard Krawiec, my first paid editor! His suggestions gave me real hope.

Finally, lots of love, hugs and kisses to my husband, Rasool, and our sons, Ali and Hassan, for their continual encouragement, support, and patience, through the years to make my dream come true.

TABLE OF CONTENTS

PREFACE

"Thank God I only have two of these!" My mammogram patient said. Boy, did she make me laugh. I had just released her right breast from the compression and still had three more pictures to take to complete her mammogram. It was early in my career as a mammographer and I was trying to find a balance of taking good films without hurting my patient. Of course after taking my films, for the patient there was still the torture of waiting to see if we were done or if more films were needed. Finally, the patient would be able to leave, without knowing the results! Lovely, isn't it!?

Later, I came across the poem, "Ode to Mammogram" by an anonymous author. I would hand the copy of the poem to my patients to read as I left to check their films adding, "It's a little R-rated, but it may make you laugh and get your mind off things. Add to it or write something yourself if you'd like to share it with others".

My intent was to ease my patient's wait and maybe have a laugh. Any cartoons or articles pertaining to mammograms, I would staple together, along with blank sheets, and offer them to my patients.

As a result, I have a collection of writings, intimate yet universal, sometimes poignant, funny and inspirational, but always wonderful.

These writings from my patients were collected before digital mammography was installed, where

I work as a mammographer, at Raleigh Radiology Cedarhurst in Raleigh, North Carolina. Digital mammography makes the whole process faster, but for the patient, the positioning, the pain, and the waiting for results, remains pretty much the same.

My patients come in all shapes and sizes. They come from different cultures and religions, a cross section of society arriving from varied responsibilities and holding different fears.

By using conversation to distract my mammogram patients, I became in awe of their stories in making their paths through life. I've gained insights, laughs, and friends in the process. The shared experience of a mammogram, the common denominator, made it all possible. I'm so grateful to be in such an important field and love what I do. Thank you ladies and men.

"ODE TO MAMMOGRAM"

For years and years they told me,
Be careful of your breasts,
Don't ever squeeze or bruise them,
And give them monthly tests.

So I heeded all their warnings
And protected them by law.
Guarded them very carefully,
And I always wore my bra.

After 30 years of astute care,
My doctor found a lump.
She ordered up a mammogram,
To look inside that bump.

"Stand up very close," she said,
as she got my boob in line.
"And, tell me when it hurts," she said.
"Ah yes! There, that's fine."

She stepped upon a peddle.
I could not believe my eyes!
A plastic plate pressed down and down,
My boob was in a vice!

My skin was stretched and stretched,
From way up under my chin.
My poor boob was being squashed,
To Swedish pancake thin.

Excruciating pain I felt,
Within its vice-like grip.

A prisoner in this vicious thing,
My poor defenseless tits!

"Take a deep breath," she said to me,
who does she think she's kidding?
My chest is mashed in her machine,
And woozy I am getting.

"There, that was good," I heard her say
as the room was slowly swaying.
"Now let's have a go at the other one."
"Lord have mercy," I was praying.

It squeezed me both from up and down,
It squeezed me from both sides,
I'll bet she's never had this done,
Not to her tender little hide!

If I had no problem when I came in,
I surely have one now.
If there had been a cyst in there,
It would have popped, ker-pow!

This machine was designed by man,
Of this I have no doubt,
I'd like to stick his balls in there,
And see how they come out!

-Anonymous

IN FEAR

"I know you've heard awful stories, but I promise you will be pleasantly surprised", I've said countless times to patients that are coming in for their first mammogram. Fear plus an empty stomach is not very conducive to a successful mammogram. Add the cooler temperature of the room and shaking and trembling come easily. Sometimes the patient looks like they're about to faint and I haven't even touched them!   The majority of the patients will say after the first film is taken, "Well, it's not as bad as I thought it would be".

I hope and trust they'll spread the word to other women.

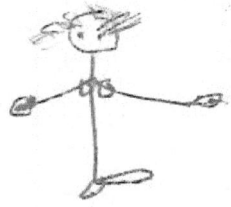

I hope this mammogram is ok because I am afraid about the cancer. Thank you. My English is very short. I am sorry.

```
To save a boob
it must be right
to squeeze it so tight.
Just hold your breath,
close your eyes and pray
```

```
everything is alright.
God bless.        Dionne M
```

It's scary, isn't it? Taking a shower and finding something in my breast that wasn't there the day before. Trying not to panic. Take it one step at a time. Then come in here with the "squisher"! Technology and language I don't understand. Just hoping that it's nothing and I can keep my breasts a while longer.

I'm 43 and this is my first time. My friends tried to really scare me but my doctor made me come anyway. I was brave, though. If only the dentist appointments could be so easy.

```
The mammogram puts you under a lot of
stress,
waiting to get results back from the test.
Hoping to hear good news,
so you won't have the blues,
after mashing your boobs.

Once a year, I have a date
to make sure you have no
lumps, or bumps,
so don't be late!
```

Why I am here today. During a self exam I felt a lump on the left. It wasn't as soft and subtle as my right breast. I asked my husband to check it out, which he kindly obliged. He agreed that it did not feel normal, so I needed to have it checked out by a trained eye! Here I sit waiting for the results, wondering my fate, but forever grateful and happy that I am at least here today! *Melissa*

To come in to get a mammogram is so scary to me because my mother died at 24 years old with breast cancer.   *Shirley*

I'm adopted and don't know what kind of things run in my family. This is a blessing to me. Yearly check-ups are a no-brainer!

Here I Sit
I sit here once again.
So many times I can't count.
But on this day, of all days
I won't forget.
It's the thirty-six years I've been
married.
So boy, what a good gift, right?
But I'm thankful to the Lord
That we ladies can come here and
Do this even though
When you leave here,
You feel like you are flat and sore.
But hoping that the end will be
A happy one.
And just waiting to find out
Is the worst.
But one thing to know, if I can be married
To the same man for thirty-six years today,
I can do this!
And I pray that
Everyone that sits in this room
Can leave with a smile in their heart.
Annette

This is my 1st mammogram and I'm 59.
  I just hope and pray that I did this on
time.
  I was scared to death when I first came
in,
  but I know God was in the room

when I entered within.

"Mammogram, oh no, not me",
that's what we always say.
We run, we hide, we panic,
and still have one someday.
Fear came from those who had the test
and it's a piercing knife.
You went and did not hear the fear
 and now it saved your life!

Men don't have large "boobs", so therefore I was not aware that
we had breast cancer. Hopefully, this is not breast cancer. Still
nervous and scared.

For piece of mind I come here year,
after year,
and I hope all will stay clear. *Melissa W*

I dreaded this so much,
 but it was really nothing.
 The fear of not knowing was worse.

I always come here crying, scared about the results I'll receive
in the mail. Today is not any different. I hope my results turn
out to be alright. I know in my heart, God is up there telling me
to have faith. *Mrs. B*

When I walked through the door,
I knew what was in store.
It came to my mind,
I hope the tech is kind.
She was, but firm
and would not let me squirm.
The room was cold
and she was so bold,
to expose them to the air,
I'd rather be anywhere.
Now, it's over, and I can breathe
and she finally lets me leave.
Oh, it wasn't so bad, except for the fear
and I will come back again next year.

Oh, the stress and the strain, anxiety.
Do I, don't I, will I, what if?
All of these questions just keep running through your mind as
you wait.

SAY CHEESE!

Mammogram. The mere mention of the word strikes fear in some women. Anxiety and dread are common responses. The women (and less frequently, men) who step into the mammogram room come for a myriad of reasons. It can be a daunting task to allow and cooperate with the mammographer to position your bare breasts for the upcoming films.

It's important to understand that the more we compress your breast, the better films we get and the less radiation you get. We want the patients to come back and get their mammograms yearly. So, I do give the patient the option to tell me to stop with the compression. This makes such a difference in the level of trust and cooperation.

If I need to compress more in order to get a good film, I will ask them. As a result, the informed patient understands the process, we work together, the films are better, as well as the experience!

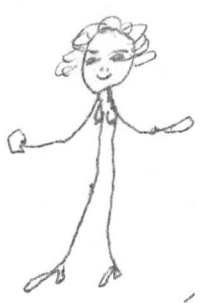

Boobs up!   *BW*

"Have you ever met someone who could breathe?" she asked with watery eyes.

It's funny when she said, "I'm going to lift your breast" and "hold your chin up". My toes curled also!   *Carol*

```
For many years I've had this done.
It really hasn't been a joy.
In fact, this machine designed by men was
really just a ploy.
But I'll keep getting this done so the
boobs will be well.
This machine, though, can go to hell!   Chris
```

```
Mammos are not fun,
Mammos are not easy.
Sometimes you want to hit the floor
for feeling queasy.
The nurse always says,
"Stand tall", "lean forward",
"look at me", "push yourself in",
and "bring your legs out".
Sometimes you look at her
and just want to shout!   Jackie G
```

For us "oldies but goldies", most of us know, "splishin and a splashin". Well, today, I was a "squishin and a squashin!"
```
From this place I'd like to get,
When she starts to squeeze my tit.
But I know it must be done,
Even tho' it is no fun.   FBS
```

I love it when they tell you "don't breathe" and "don't move". How could you?

Because of my voluminous breasts, I once again smashed my face on the equipment. There was no where else for it to go! Has anyone other than me wondered what would happen if the power went off suddenly, with one breast clamped down tighter than imaginable?! I hope I never find out! Thanks for laughing with me.

Nervous was I, when I arrived.
All the haunting tales filled my mind.
I prayed before I entered the room
to face the "breast-pancake-machine's
music tune.
As it pressed down, my nipple almost
popped!
But just as I was about to scream, the
mashing stopped. *Shamika*

It was soooo much fun, I'll be braless for a few days!

As my face is smashed against this wonderful machine, I rationalize my dilemma. My twin sister and I are sharing boobs that were meant for one person!
Yeah, I was feeling like a model, too, laughing all the way! My poor, tattooed, boob sure looked different all flattened out!
Press! Press!
Smash! Smash!
Hold it or my boob may go woosh!!

They say, "relax", "stand here", "don't breathe or move", and "relax". Not so easy to do while your breast is getting smashed.

It is more uncomfortable than painful and worth every second.

"Stand straight". "Move forward".

"Are you okay?" "Yes".
"Don't breathe". "Hold it". "Okay". "Don't move..."Let's do the other one".
"You are all done".

Great to know everything is okay.
It was worth the squeezing, mashing.

Well, they sure look big on film!

G-rrr means, "STOP!"

Hey, if I scream, she might smash them more!

They're grapes, they're gonna pop!!

You don't know how big your breasts really are until they are smashed under a plate glass! I was thinking mine won't go past the diagram. So much for my thinking, they looked bigger than the plate!

She squished
the twins,
my boobs!
How quickly I forgot there were 4 films needed. What comfort in hearing no more films needed!

Just one question, are they touching my knees, or does it just feel that way? *Kim*

Keep going, keep going, the flatter the better.
A wonderful radiograph at last.

There's no needles, probes, or hanging
tubes,
Just the machine, a tech, me and my boobs.
The boobs are pushed and pulled and
thoroughly mashed.
But after some time I'm out of here in a
flash!

This was no fun, it was not nice.
My hooters squished within a vice.
But when she let me go, hooray!
And that's all that I have to say.   *Sally*

My breasts are big. Still are after coming in here!
I found out after all I had nothing to fear.
My husband will be glad there's still something left to feel.

Pressed, stressed, and strained,
Is the name of this game.
I turn left, I turn right.
I pray my results are cheerful and bright.
I'm treated well and I feel great.
Getting this mammogram is for my sake.
This is an important test.
We all dislike it, I confess,
but I know it is for the best. God bless.

Just think, when I arrived, I thought I was having a bad day.
Who knew that I was actually driving myself to a destination,
wherein, someone was going to torture me by squeezing the life
out of my boobs! I'm sitting here waiting for her to tell me I
can go. "Psyche", she's back, and needs one more film!

Think of it this way, the day will be all downhill from here!

My aunt-in-law just had a breast removed two months ago. Self examination and this monstrous machine is a blessing. "Just a little pressure here", and "turn this way, please", is all okay. The words, "move your stomach, please" is what scares me. All in all it's okay. Every woman should have a mammogram day!
Bernice

I've waited many years to get boobies. I had them when I came here today. I've been told that "having them" makes it hurt less than "not having them". Now they're flat from being squeezed! Water bras are looking pretty good to me right now while I wait for mine to bounce back! ***KL***

My breasts are so small,
They hardly fit on the plate at all.
So, that's it. A pull, a yank, a gentle tug.
A yearly check will do.
What great words all through!
It helps! ***CA***

On the way home I will need to stop and purchase a new bra. I never noticed if they stocked "pancake-flat-double A's! They could be hard to locate. Wish me luck. ***Nancy***

```
A procedure said to be simple and no pain
at all,
actually sent me speeding woozily down the
hall.
I could barely get to my vehicle to get
home safe and sound.
Of course you can tell I'm stretching the
truth all the way around.
```

Something should be devised so that man can share in this delightful experience! Weird, isn't it? How your boobs look like an emptied wallet afterwards?! ***Betty***

23

My perky little boobs perk no more.
This monster-mash-machine has mashed them
toward the floor. *Kathy*

The Mammoscam:
It's not that I mind the pain you see,
it's just that it's so humiliating to
me.
To stand there with them out in all
their glory,
but that's not the end of the story.
"Step up close, no closer, no closer
still".
"Ok, right there".
"I'll let this down some", she says,
but not of course to where
it keeps going and going and going.
You think it's going to pop!
The next thing you know,
you are seeing stars!
Oh, can you please stop?
"I'm sorry it hurts", she says so
sweetly,
"but now I have to do the other
one",
as you sigh deeply.
It all starts again,
and the words "it'll only hurt a
bit",
echo in my mind.
The man who came up with this cruel
punishment,
telling us, "It's for our good",
I would like to find.
So to all my sisters in pain,
remember,
it's for the cause.

And it's only the beginning, for we still
have to look forward to
"mentalpause".

SIZE MATTERS

Large breasted women versus small breasted women. The large breasted women many times say, "How do you do those little ones?" The small breasted women many times say, "How do you do those big ones?" Well, I tell them, they can all be challenging. It may be a little more difficult to get a tiny breast up on the plate and you may need to take more films for a large breasted woman.

There's a lot of large breasted women who would rather be small, and there's also a lot of small breasted women who would rather be large. Too bad there isn't a sharing system.

No matter what size breast you have, there's one thing all breasts have in common, they're all different! I almost wish I had done this job as a teenager, because I've learned that there's a whole range of normal and we're all okay!

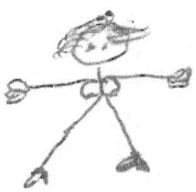

God bless these little tits. They are so small, they couldn't be stretched.

You're naked in front of a complete stranger and your boobs feel like they're ten feet long! *Elizabeth*

```
This is the only time
 having small breasts was so bad.
Boy, if they were bigger
 I couldn't imagine the pain I would've
had!
God Bless!   Kianna
```

I always dread the mammogram. Maybe that's because I have a D-cup and sooo much boob to press! But this time it was not so bad. *Laurie*

Thank the Lord for bras with wire in them to hold up my saggy boobs.

```
'Twas the day of my mammo and all was a
clatter.
But lo and behold she did not bring the
platter!
I am so self conscious because they're so
huge.
The technology is one we all can't refuse!
Good luck and God bless our technicians!
PD
```

Our sympathy to Dolly Parton. God bless those ladies who only have "skeeter" bites for breasts!

If you get nervous about this procedure remember this:
-Large breasts are a pain in the rear as we get older, they ruin your posture.
-They give you neck, shoulder, and back pain
-You can't swing a golf club or tennis racket because you're too busy pulling them out of your arm pits!
-Bras are expensive.
etcetera, etcetera.
If your man wants big boobs, get him a bra and put a pound of sugar in each bra cup. Have him wear it around until he starts whining about it. You'll probably only have to wait about fifteen minutes! If he doesn't get it, get rid of him!

If only a miracle bra pulled and squished like this, I might have had some cleavage!   *Elsie P*

This was on my 40th birthday card from my best friend since kindergarten. Boy, have we watched each other change!
    "Do your boobs hang low?
      Do they wobble to and fro?
      Can you tie'em in a knot?
      Can you tie'em in a bow?"
Of course, the answer to all of the above is yes! But I guess they are healthy. Oh, on the inside of the card, it said, "Have a "perky(less) birthday!"   Keep smiling!   *Susan*

My breast used to be small.
Now I wear a double D and that's not all.
They are like a pancake and flat.   *Bennett*

What a pleasant visit to this clinic! I've always been self-conscious about my flat chest. But today you squeezed, pushed, and pulled, to put something on the tray. Suddenly I realized that I have breasts! They were there all the time, but just hiding from me. Thank you.

I guess you've seen it all!

Those of you who think having big, plump, breasts is great, I'm sure you have more problems when visiting Susan and her machine. I get to enjoy the fact that my breasts are now like elastic bands. They seem to work with the machine, s-t-r-e-t-c-h! *Bettie*

Can't believe it!
My breasts are so small,
they mashed down to cow tit size!
What a miracle!

There was a time in my life when my breasts were very small. When I had a mammogram, the lady giving me my mammogram and I would try our best to find something to x-ray! As I have gotten much, much, older, I now have boobies that can be x-rayed without much tugging and pulling. I am very proud of them today! So you small breasted ladies, there is hope. I always thought that if I did have a lump, it would be very obvious!

A friend of mine is a plastic surgeon. One day I asked what test he used to determine if a woman needed a breast lift. He said to stand tall, with good posture and chest out. If you can hold a pencil under your breast you may be a candidate. I said, "pencil, heck, I can hold a two liter bottle of Coke!

I am just thankful that she found something to squash, being one of those small breasted gals.

It's the only time I'm glad I have large, floppy, breasts.

Having been flat-chested all my life, I heard jokes about how would I get a mammogram. I now say that the only good part of the middle age spread is some of it goes to the boobs!   *BME*

```
"A" cup, "B" cup, "C" cup, "D",
whatever cup you happen to be.
Mammograms are a must
Even with a big bust,
Unless you are a tree...
```
Eileen R

"Nanny, why are nanny's boobs down here and mommy's are up there?" "Well, sweet child, you don't know what the word gravity means. Someday you will."   *3 year old to a 60 year old.*

I was so "top heavy" in my twenties that my brother would tease me by saying I defied the laws of gravity to be standing upright. Thank God for breast reductions. There should be a breast bank for donations to small breasted women!   *Joanne C*

I'm glad to have boobs to squeeze.

OH, WHAT A FEELING!

Pain.

Okay, there's certain times of the month I wouldn't come near this machine myself. I find myself cringing in sympathy with my patients on those days. Also, if I've been drinking too many sweet teas or ice coffees, I'm grateful it's not mine under the compression paddle. But otherwise, I think it goes pretty quick.

Tattoos. I've seen an increase of tattoos on my patients through the years. Like breast implants, it crosses all ages and occupations! I would think getting a tattoo must be painful, more so than getting a mammogram. So, when I have a patient with tattoos, who is scared of the mammogram, I find that hard to understand.

I've heard some great stories connected to tattoos from my patients, but this is one of my favorites:

My patient had a friend that had breast cancer. She had accompanied her on her chemo and radiation treatments, shaved her hair in solidarity, and when her friend had passed the five year mark, breast cancer free, they both went to get a tattoo to celebrate!

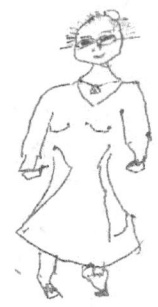

Compared to childbirth and an abscessed tooth, this is a piece of cake! Thankful for the opportunity.

The machine is strong as can be,
It takes pictures and "they" want to yell,
"Don't squeeze! It hurts! Slow down!"
They say, "I'm not squash!"   *RJS*

On a bright, Monday morning, go and get your boobs squished.
Great.

```
The skin is not tight and my boobs are
sore.
When this mammogram is over, they will
hit the floor.
A line is needed, instead of a bra, to hold
them up as you can see.
I was mashed so hard, I had to pee!
```

Well, all I can say is "Ouch!" "Damn it!" "Get the ### off of me!" Excuse my French, "###!"

I can only hope the machine gets a good picture because I'd hate to have to repeat this. If not, I pray it wasn't because it didn't squish "lefty" enough. It was with my last breath that I conjured up the command to "stop!".

This will be a good reason to get them kissed later, not groped, grabbed or sucked!

It wasn't too bad, just felt like a tire ran over my boob! *DGM*

My mom always said she had perky breasts until she started having them smooshed once a year. She was blessed never to have breast cancer. It's a small price to pay to prevent something more serious. But really, do we have to get them as flat as a pancake to check?

If I moved now, I think I'd rip them off! *Jeanne*

```
The  last  time  I  felt  such  pain  was  one  of
great  worth.
The  last  time  I  felt  such  pain  was  when  I
last  gave  birth!
P.S.  But  then  I  got  the  epidural.
```

I hope you did not do like me and promise your husband a romantic night at home .I did this before I came here, not knowing of the pain.
If he gets satisfaction tonight, he will do it alone!

I've got big boobs and the only time I regret it is when I come here! Can you say "ooowwwww!" *Amy*

I'm thirty six. I came in for my first one and the nurse said, "Oh, since you have tattoos, you will be fine." It still hurt. Have a good day.

33

We have it done every year but the pain is still there. I wonder if large breasted women hurt as much as small breasted women.

Lordy! Lordy! Have mercy, I'm glad this is done only once a year! **Donna P**

At least I don't have to bend over and cough!

If only I could breathe while this was going on and hold my belly in at the same time!

This machine squeezes me like my ex-husband.

Oh, no! My small ones necessitated pulling down my chin!

I was asked to not swing at the technician if she compressed me too much. My response was that it would be difficult since she had me between a rock and a hard place!

Thank God my husband is not a breast man. He won't see these for awhile.

Just remember ladies, it's not as bad as labor pains. We can call it the "Squish-O-Matic""! If it helps, why not?

For a brief moment you feel like they might actually break! Other than that, I always encourage other women to get this done! Too bad these things aren't detachable.

And they wonder why it takes us forever to want to schedule these.

It felt like my boob was sucked out/off like a vacuum cleaner to your skin. Weird more than painful. Better than the alternative. Though, I would like to see a man go through this!

Dear Lord, I asked, why me?
She mashed my boobs, so hard, I could not see.
The pain was tremendous.
This I will surely remember.
The pain left quickly.
I'm so glad I don't have to do this weekly!
God bless all who read this. *VAR*

Thank goodness it's done by a female,, it's so much more comfortable. Hey, between this and a pelvic exam, there's no contest!!

She's got me all prepped for the dentist now. I'm sure he's going to hurt a lot worse.

One question, are we having fun yet? Ain't it great to be a woman! Men just couldn't do all that we do.

It's not that bad. They bounce right back to their perfect shape. *Donna L*

Today was a good day for me and my boobs. My husband squeezes them a whole lot harder. *Monica*

It wasn't bad at all, especially compared to the horrible e-mails I've read. I'd do this over a pap smear any day!

It is uncomfortable, but hey, it's important. It's not as bad as being in labor. So grin and bear it! Thank you. Merci! Abiento! *Linda.*

Whew! Technology leaves a lot to be desired. Love and laugh often! God, I love being a woman.

Had a wonderful time. How often do you get to have your breast fondled and squeezed by rubber and machine?! Thanks, **Cori**

Ladies, relax, it's a great feeling. Take a deep breath. Hold it. Smile. **M Evans**

All the pressing is worth it to screen for cancer and catch it early! It was not so bad. But I'll wait a year before I do it again! **MM**

YA GOTTA LAUGH!

The title for this book came from one of my first patients as a mammographer. Trust me, there are many women out there that should be stand-up comics. The mammogram became their material. Many times I had to try and be stern to have them stop laughing, so there wouldn't be any motion on the film. At the same time I would be struggling to stifle myself so as to not restart the laughter...at least until the exposure was done!

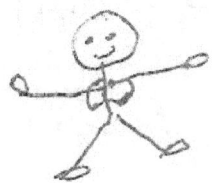

I always appreciate the choice in attractive gowns. Aqua is one of my favorite colors. I was successful in tying it together, but as usual, had one tie left over. Why are there three ties?

Thanks for a "mammorable" experience! *Virginia*

A mammogram squashed
Your breast so flat,
You can mail them
Like an envelope!

This could be the highlight of my day. I'm getting poked and pinched at both ends today!

I'm fine. I'm fine. I know that I am fine. But if not, please take them both off, so I can get the set I have always dreamed of! *SH*

I am glad to come but happier to leave! I love my tits! Great for nursing my four children and for great sex with my sweetie!

I'm all flab, so the test didn't hurt at all! *Marg*

I always look forward to my regular boob-o-gram, when they make my cup into a saucer! *Frieda*

But on the other hand, my dear,
once squeezed and squashed, I need
not fear.
My lovely breasts are back to normal
and I'll look quite sexy in my black,
velvet formal. *Elizabeth A*

Boobs, boobs, boobs!
What can ya do, do, do?

As I sit here thinking of my breasts
I think having none would be the best.
But then I consider the lowly sow
Who has seven more than the lucky cow!

Mammogram is "breast origami"! Shape up for the fight against breast cancer. Can they do a swan?!
I think I'm at the wrong office. It's my knees! My knees, that need attention! Thanks!

When asked what my plans for the day were, I quipped, "the twins are getting photographed today!" *Peg*

If only my boobies would stay up the way she put them!

I forgot how strange these positions are! They would make a great abstract painting!
D Fitzgerald

During the early days when the wringer washer was in use, women's tits accidentally got caught in the wringer and caused a lot of pain. Today the torture is part of our annual health exam and is performed by appointment and is not free! We have come a long way! **Nahid**

Definitely created by a man!

So were panty hose!

Well, I'm convinced a woman invented the necktie!

My deceased mother-in-law once told me that after forty, it's just patch, patch, patch! Thanks for helping keep my breasts patched and healthy.

Now I know the origin of the expression "booby trap".

If my fiancé knew that a machine was taking pictures of my breast, he would want to buy a digital camera and take pictures every year for HIS records. **Sheila J**
When I come here, I tell my friends, "it's time for the girls to have their picture taken."

What does an 80 year old woman have between her breasts that a 20 year old woman doesn't? Her belly button. **(a 70 yr old patient)**

Ladies, go get your mammies "grammed"!   *SM*

I'll go home tonight and tell my husband, "Honey, I don't need you tonight, I had a mammogram today!

I'm just glad I only have to have one squeezed!   *EMS*

I wonder why God makes them grow
when we get old and cold.
I have no husband, just some "grands",
and if I might say, the boobs are gone too!
I have a request, I'd like, of which I feel is true.
Let me shed the boobs, dear God, and
please grow a new set of teeth!!

If women were given breasts for feeding babies, why do men have them?

I'm 86 years old and told my doctor I was just too old to be taking a mammogram. She just looked at me and said, "Oh, no! As long as you have boobs, you have mammograms. If you wake up one morning and don't have any, then we'll stop". So here I am.   *Virgina*

NOT SO BAD

There are plenty of patients that don't understand all the moaning and groaning about the mammogram. They don't find it so uncomfortable.

Now, for those patients that do find the mammogram painful, there are some helpful ideas.

Patients have discovered that cutting down on caffeine has lessened their breast pain. Caffeine is found in coffee, tea, sodas, and even chocolate. Chocolate, of course, is too important to cut out of our diet.

Also, scheduling the mammogram four to five days after menstruation has begun is helpful.

The benefits of Vitamin E and other vitamins you may hear of combating breast pain need to be discussed with your doctor.

Bottom line, patients have to decide how important is this once a year exam, and then the decision is a "no brainer".

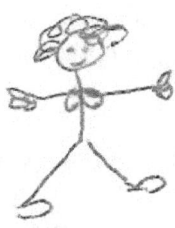

I knew pain was near

```
but it was all a piece of cake,
especially knowing this is for my sake!
```

Glad it's over, not too painful. The boob was flat. Hope it puffs
up again.

I really didn't feel like I closed my breasts in the refrigerator
door. Small breasts rule!

This is the one time having larger breasts pays off. It's getting
easier and easier. There's not as much pain or pinching.

Squeeze away. This is nothing compared to childbirth.

The procedure was not as bad as worrying about it. Thanks for
keeping me healthy. *Elaine*

No pain lasts forever, we just think it does. *Martha*

So glad it's not a man that's doing the exam! *Jen*

Not bad at all. Glad it's over because I am a big chicken!
Janice

This was my first time. I was pretty scared but it was no pain at
all. Never believe what you hear because it's different strokes
for different folks. And it didn't take long at all. Be blessed.
Aida

Not much pain. Good news please!
Mary M
```
A squeeze, not a slice.
Once a year and you're done.
Good results.
```

Now have some fun! *Suzanne*

I was told before arriving to expect the same feeling as though the "garage door had squashed my breasts". I was pleasantly surprised that it was nowhere near as uncomfortable as I had expected. I wouldn't say that this would be something that I would add to my daily regimen but it's worth it for the peace of mind afterwards.

I can take it…I can take it…I can take it…I can take it…Can I breathe now? Well, that wasn't so bad!

It was not an unbearable experience. Before I knew it, it was over! I now am feeling healthier just for doing it!

```
I've heard so many stories
and they all were simply untrue.
Because this procedure was merely
uncomfortable,
And now I feel as good as new.
```

I am 89 years old. This is the first mammogram I have ever had. Not bad.

Hopefully a little pain today will save a lot of pain tomorrow.

What was the big deal? Even with a lump and sore breast, it was painless. After childbirth, pain is definitely relative.
Anne

I thought they would smash them flat and they would never spring back! It's not as bad as I thought or heard.
I have a friend that said it hurt so much when she got her mammogram that she would never get another. I can stand the

43

pain for awhile if it would keep me from having worse pains like cancer, later on. There has to be a little rain with the sunshine. Chins up, ladies.

Sure it's uncomfortable for a few seconds but it beats the heck out of the alternative. *Linda*

Thank God for this wonderful, although temporarily, painful test. One year ago, a cyst was found deep, too deep to feel. I now know and am more aware of what I need to do to keep an eye on it. I now take better care of myself!

For years I've been told that a mammogram would hurt. This machine was designed to save our lives.
So ladies, no matter how long we put it off,
there is no need to hide. I did it, I made it, with no problem at all. For real, ladies, it wasn't bad and I had a ball! I waited until I was thirty-seven years old. It's over now and time for me to put back on my clothes.

This is temporary. What you might find…might not be.

We need to count our blessings. Compared to having surgery or even death, what is a mammogram? So let us all be thankful. *Rev. J D*

A little pain is worth the loads of relief you feel
when you get the report, "normal". What a load off your mind. And if not normal, thank God for a machine that can help find the smallest problem and go get it fixed. It is worth the small inconvenience.

For a woman who doesn't have a lot of boob tissue, you sure found something to squish!! This little procedure wasn't sooo bad!! The "girls" and I thank you!

Now I know what a cubed steak feels like! Seriously, though, not so bad. Certainly, it's a huge head and shoulders above the possible alternatives! JUST DO IT!

A moment of discomfort for a year of well being and early detection. It's well worth the moment for the piece of mind!

I can think of so many more pleasant things to do with my time, but isn't wonderful to have this test that takes so little time and saves so lives.

Let's consider this: mammogram pain compared to the pain of breast cancer.

Thank God for tests that make us aware of any problems we may have. It only hurts for a little while.   *DJB*

The peace of mind will be well worth it. I avoided this for years. The inevitable wasn't as bad as I'd heard. But glad I won't be here for a year.

A little bit of pain is nothing compared to the relief from anxiety you get with good results!   *Sharon*

All the fuss about this scared me to death. This was not bad at all. Go ladies, you can do it.

At 42 years old, I didn't realize I had such big boobs. It really wasn't that bad.

Ladies, it didn't hurt at all and I'm a C-cup! Thank God for this machine. It has helped save lives and one day it could be mine.

This procedure is necessary. Have you had children? Nothing, almost nothing, can compare with childbirth pain. The pain of childbirth is worth it! The pain of a mammogram is worth it! *Delores*

It's better to be able to have a mammogram than to NOT be able to. *Jackie*

```
I guess it's worth the price you pay,
when nothings what they find.
Now I can go another year
with total peace of mind.   Donna H
```

All I can say is, I'm thankful that we have mammograms. Years ago they didn't. I wonder how many women died of breast cancer? And did they know it was breast cancer? Even though the mammogram is uncomfortable, it could save my life! I'm lucky to have the "squeeze"!

A slight discomfort but what a wonderful feeling afterwards to know if something shows up, you got it early. *Brenda K*

I'm twenty two and this is my first time. To make matters worse, I'm on my period, so my breasts are more sensitive. But honestly, it wasn't as bad as I imagined. It goes pretty quick.

Keep smilin'! We can endure any pain for a limited time. Think about people who are in pain 24/7. *Barbara*

Oh, how lucky we are to have such testing! What's a minute of squeezing if it saves lives. Squeeze away!

Every year when I have a mammogram, it looks to me to be a very simple visit. I try to work with the nurse and I make myself ready to get any results. *HB*

I am grateful to be alive and well. True this is an inconvenience but it's worth it. Life is short enough, so I'm going to enjoy it for as long as I can.

IT'S PERSONAL/TESTIMONIES

Zari was a good friend whom I met when our family first moved to Raleigh, North Carolina. She bravely fought breast cancer for 14 years. She continually stayed positive and spiritually strong. I learned so much from her.

I'm very grateful for the few times I was able to accompany her to chemotherapy appointments. Of course, that was followed by lunch out, discovering new foods together! Sometimes we would meet up with old friends of hers that were anxious to stay a part of Zari's life.

Zari encouraged her husband, Mark, and their daughter, Katie, to pursue their interests and activities and found great joy listening to their stories. Mark and Zari would travel, visiting relatives and friends for happy occasions and even made a glorious trip to Italy! They went out, socialized, and enjoyed life together as a couple and as a family. Mark, Zari, and Katie were there for each other, always.

Zari had a great many supportive and prayerful friends that kept her occupied with lunches, birthdays, and other activities. She and some of these girlfriends had a last wonderful, memorable, trip to the beach!

Zari was so amazing. Up until her death, she fought her breast cancer by living life to the fullest, laughing and loving.

Mammography is very personal to me.

Gwen was an old friend from my hometown, St. Louis, Missouri. She bravely fought breast cancer for 13 years.

Gwen was a clinical research coordinator working with breast cancer clinical trials recruiting women. She even became a minister to be able to help patients coping with all kinds of serious illnesses which unfortunately she knew too well.

Up until her death, she was trying to develop a non-profit organization to help women going through the chemo and radiation process to pay their bills, gas, and any other needs women have while trying to fight the breast cancer battle. Gwen definitely would've approved of the Caring Community Foundation. She was so strong, full of faith, and determined to win the battle while helping others. She really tried to make a difference in women's lives.

Sisters Network, Inc., is an important national African American breast cancer survivorship organization which, at one time, Gwen was president of the St. Louis, Missouri chapter.

My friend lived and breathed the struggle against breast cancer for her and others on a daily basis.

Gwen kept most of her struggles from her mother, Bennie and her son, Geoffrey. She was a force in action that her family, friends, and colleagues loved and prayed for always. California was the scene for a last wonderful trip with her sister, Pam, with lots of shopping bags in hand!

Yes, mammography is very personal to me. Look around yourself. Breast cancer has touched all of us in one way or another.

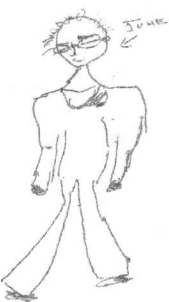

I am a 3 year survivor from breast cancer. It was found in this room by a mammogram at an early, early, stage. It works! Spread the word. This machine, this staff, and God, all work together. *LPRH*

Don't be afraid of the mammograms even though they squish you to an acorn. My cancer was found this way and now I'm okay. At least they only get to squish one now! Bless the mammogram. *CAS*

I saw a woman I worked with die because she was afraid to go to the doctor after finding a lump. A year later, she had a radical mastectomy and never won the fight. Knowledge gives you power and choices.

Here I am today,
a place I didn't want to be.
But with a sister just diagnosed, I have to
be sure,
it also isn't me!

So squeeze and flatten my little boobs
on and on.
A little calmer and wiser,
and in the know.   *LA*

Ladies, just do it! You will not regret it. I have lost four
friends. What's a little pain in exchange for your life?
Melinda M

A family history of cancer, then your daughter develops breast
cancer and has a mastectomy. You know the mammogram truly
has a place in your life. Four years later my daughter is doing
great! *DT*

My best friend has had mastectomies and now is cancer free. I
always encourage friends to have this done. I wonder if those
giving them have it done also?! *Nancy L*

This saved my sister when she was 51. I had breast cancer in
January, 2001. My cancer was so small it could not be felt. But
with everything pulled from my back through the vise, the
tumor was detected on the mammogram. . Get it checked out
now! That's the least you deserve after that vise job. I'm doing
great now. Thanks to God and medical personnel! *Eunice*

My sister, Ellen, wasn't as fortunate as most of us. She had
cancer, but thank God, mammogram caught it early! She's fine.
Joanne

As uncomfortable as they can be, I understand their necessity. My mother, a 12 year survivor. My mother-in-law, a 10 year survivor. My sister-in-law, a 4 year survivor. All due to early detection. I shutter to think what life would be like without these wonderful people to learn, laugh, and play with! *Sherry L*

This is easy compared to a lumpectomy. It's all worth it for the peace of mind.   Thanks, *Elaine*

Having had breast cancer in 1992, I feel the expression "the good ol' days" are now! New technology and attitudes professionals now have to diagnose are encouraging to us with this horrid disease. I am ever so grateful for the kind words and news of discoveries in fighting this disease and the hope for each and all.   *S Ford*

My friend, Sandra, lost her fight with breast cancer just a few months before her 54th birthday. Is there any better reason for me to have a mammogram? I consider this procedure my living tribute to her each year. It's been light years now. God, I miss her. PS. I can't leave on a "downer", so I'll add a favorite quote: "small busted women, (that's me) have big hearts". *Elaine*

Thank God for mammograms. I am a 5 year survivor. Who knows if I could have been here to get my boobs squished one more time?

Cancer survivor. Diagnostic mammogram. Thank God I only have one of these!

As a cancer survivor, a mammogram does not hurt like it used to. A mammogram or a "dirtnap", what a choice! I choose the mammogram.   Thanks, *Annette*

For Leigh, she will be a survivor.

I dreaded coming in today. The mammogram is usually painful for my small breasts! Today wasn't so bad. I wonder if the last lady was masochistic!! My sister comes soon, she's had one breast removed. I hope her results will be ok and mine, too. She's the most upbeat person I know who has lost a breast.

Big machines like these are a major step in detecting any unforeseen problems. Faced with many uncertainties, I'd get mashed boobs any day. Breast cancer has taken several of my family members over the years. I really pray that someday research will get a cure.

I have a dear friend who had breast cancer. Going through it with her made me aware how important this test is. You would not believe her pain.

It all started because I got busty. For a skinny person this was really important. A grapefruit-sized tumor was found. They gave me three months to live and I am still here. The mammogram is my friend/foe. Without it I would have never known. I beat the odds and survived. Peace and sunny days to come. *Evelyn*

I am very confident having a mammogram. I lost my best friend to breast cancer at age 33. I am now 50! What a long way mammography has come. So little pain and so much to gain. Peace of mind is worth a million. My friend would be 50, June 28th. Happy birthday, Sue.
Kathy P

Please get your mammogram each year, they can save your life. It saved my mother!! Thank you, *Doreen*

I have family who are survivors due to early detection! I'm glad my Labradors don't have to get mammograms. Eight times each dog, yikes! Plus, they're uninsured dependents!

A lump on my friend did appear.
She said, "It's just a bump, my dear".
"Oh, to the doctor you must go".
With stubbornness, she politely said,
"No".
I stood my ground and did insist.
On calling the doctor, my eyes a mist.
Sure enough my fears came true.
My friend had cancer and I was blue.
Four years have passed and all is fine.
Thank God for miracles, He is divine!
Lynn R.

The press is uncomfortable but I thank God for it. Had it been used in the 1970's, some people would have been helped...my mother. *Frannie*

After watching some of my friends suffer with breast cancer, I look forward to getting close to this nice machine. Sisterly

A mammogram saved my life. The little white spot was like a tiny star burst. But this cute little star burst was"in-situ cancer". It was less than Stage 1 but it could have grown to Stage 1 or more by my next mammogram. I only have a minor scar on my left breast. Early detection prevented the loss of my breast. God has blessed all of us with this uncomfortable test. Please take it. If not for yourself, for your family and friends. *DCP*

I'm so thankful for this test. It can be so helpful to keep us informed of the unknown. Many of my friends and my sister have breast cancer. I thank God that they had their mammograms done faithfully and did their monthly breast checks. Keep up the good work.

I have an aunt who is a breast cancer survivor thanks to early screening. However, I lost a dear friend to breast cancer at age 30. I pray for a cure.

Having lost two friends, too young, to this disease, I count myself lucky to have screenings only!
I've lost 8 relatives to the big C
and this year, 5 dear friends.
These lumps and bumps
will not get me.
That's how my poem ends!   *Anita*

I lost my friend ironically this morning to breast cancer. She has fought it courageously as it moved to other parts of her body. She was a vivacious woman that would tell everyone to get their mammograms and do breast exams. This is a tribute to you. I love you, JoAnn. See you in heaven.   Love, *Cindy*
I watched a friend die of cancer a couple of years ago. Being more careful might have saved her life. The pain and "sticking" is a small price to pay to avoid that particular terror.

I had a breast removed at age 40 due to early stage breast cancer. I'm now 56 with no recurrence and in pretty good health. Mammograms are necessary!

May 2002, my doctor called and asked if my husband could come to his office so that my biopsy could be discussed. I asked him right there on the phone if I had breast cancer. No member of my family has ever had breast cancer. We went in to see him. He explained that the small spot on my mammogram was cancerous. Black women have a low rate of survival from breast cancer. After telling him all the things that I would not do to live for five more years, the doctor informed us that the cancer had been detected early and had not invaded any other area of my breast. Surgery would remove it all. That was 32 months ago. The treatments were energy stealing. I had lymphedema. Lymphoderma therapy relieved the swelling and pain with massages and wraps. I'm feeling great and very blessed. Early detection, diet, exercise, and a loving, caring, family has helped me to get back to a normal, secure, life. Thanks to Raleigh Radiology Cedarhurst for that early detection through my annual mammogram. ***Devah***

Early detection is an absolute must for us. My sister had breast cancer and it was found too late. So thank God for this process and let's keep coming to have it done! ***BMC***

My best friend just had a double mastectomy. I was the one who pushed her into her first mammogram. Now, I'm glad I did and I'm here like clockwork!
Although breast cancer hasn't hit my direct family yet, I have lost many relatives on both sides of the family and husband's side. My concerns now are for my mother and daughters.

Explanations of what you're doing and why, makes the whole process easier.

I'm so thankful to God and my savior Jesus for giving me 61 years of life. This test helped save my life. I had a mastectomy last year and the only way it was found was by a mammogram. If this test was created by a man, I still appreciate it. Thanks be to God.

Piece of cake. In August, my good friend from childhood will be dead from breast cancer for four years. She fought it for 10 years. She left behind a four year old son. I hear her words, "do it yearly" and I comply. In memory of Gwen.

Freedom from the fear of having cancer is what the mammogram means to me. My husband lost a niece to breast cancer and I think of her every year when I get my mammogram. She would be proud to know that she is thought of in this special way. *Nancy*

My DCIS was caught by mammography and I had a lumpectomy right away. Had it not been for my mammogram, this lump wouldn't have been detected for many years. I'm only 43 years old. *CW*

In July 1999, I was diagnosed with breast cancer through diagnostic mammogram, and had chemo and radiation. I'm thankful to come in and get "squashed" again. I have learned much and am grateful for today. So smile even if it hurts. It's better than the alternative. Be of good courage for the Lord is mighty in power, love and grace. *Louise*
My sister has just gone through her first chemo treatment because of breast cancer. It's something no one should have to

ever go through. Thank God for mammograms. The slight pain is nothing compared to what you could go through! ***Billie B***

Today I can add another note in my journal, from July 28, 2000, when I got the diagnosis of breast cancer. What a gift to receive one day before your birthday, 7-29-?!! Bet you thought I was telling you my age. Whatever the outcome of today, I can live with it after the initial shock. The power of prayer and faith, and the patience and compassion of your provider. Thanks, ***Mary G***

Please pray for my sister-in-law. She has breast cancer. She is going thru chemo, surgery, radiation and reconstruction. She is only 38! She never had a mammogram. Thanks, ***Jane W.***

Ladies, I just want to say that once you hit 40, you seem to start falling apart! Tomorrow is my 43rd birthday and hopefully I'll see my 50th! My mother is a breast cancer survivor. Get those mammograms done, ladies, it's worth a little pain. Could save your life!

My only breast is so long and fat.
I just throw it over my shoulder, onto my back!
My only breast is so long and fat.
I have it over my shoulder and a pillow for my back! ***MRT***

Mammograms

I never had a mammogram until my doctor
felt a lump.
On the road of life I was about to hit a
bump.
I was too young to even start, not yet the
big 4-0.
But off for a mammogram, quickly I did go.
They called it "diagnostic" instead of
just screening.
Since I was new at this that really had no
meaning.
I soon found out that it meant they were
concerned.
Mammograms and ultrasounds, I had a lot to
learn.
I trusted all these people; I knew they had
the answers.
Thank God for the mammogram, it discovered
I had cancer.
The mammo found it early, while it was very
small.
That's why I'm still here to write this
poem at all.
So go for your mammogram, it's only once a
year.
I know it can be painful and it raises lots
of fear.
The alternative is worse, you might not
find out in time.
EARLY DETECTION SAVES LIVES (although it
doesn't rhyme)   *Julie*

KEEP THE FAITH

Raleigh, the capital of North Carolina, has people from all over the world, many transplants from other states, as well as native North Carolinians. This makes for an intersection of all kinds of religious faiths and personal spiritual paths, that arrive for a mammogram. I've listened to their words as they walked into my room and upon leaving. Similarities that tie all the beliefs together is the strength and fearlessness with which they face the unknown.

I think you will find while you read the words below that no matter the patients background, their words will sound familiar to you.

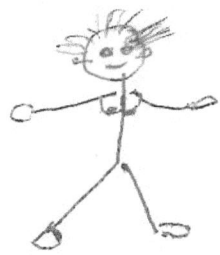

Dear Lord, I know you are with me. Please take this test into your hands. What will be, will be. But I know you love me and are in control for me. *CRH*

Fun, fun, fun.
Nothing to fear.
Remember fear knocked at the door,
faith answered. *Joyce W.*

Whatever we go through, always remember God is in the experience. You are never alone. So just take your mind off the problem.

Fear is always trying to keep us trapped. Remember there is nothing too hard for God. Smile.

A nice lady greets you with a smile, offers you a gown and a wipe. You undress and go through the process with the thoughts of every woman before you. I decided to let God do his work and stay out of it! **RS**

Since I put myself in the hand of the Lord, I have no fear. God bless.

When I rose up this morning,
It wasn't by my plan.
I somewhat feared, almost dreaded,
The thought of a mammogram.
But as God always will spring blessings
upon his people,
I busied along and made ready for the test.
Keeping now faith to the very best.
My Lord, My savior, Jesus Christ.

Life is a precious gift to be used in the service of the Lord. The mammogram procedure is what it is, a time to reflect on the miracle of life.
Linda S

I was called back for a second test for the first time in eight years. I came in with my shield of faith knowing God is with me. I trust everything will be fine either way. Have faith, not fear. **Julia**

I know that Allah will take care of me today and always. I am in his hands.

God said in his word he would never leave us or forsake us. Whatever the outcome of these pinching tests, He will lead the way and be with us always. I have nothing to fear.   *Sandi L*

This was my fourth mammogram and I can surely say I felt it was my best. Maybe losing weight made the skin tissue feel less painful. I'm not worried because I know the Lord wouldn't give me any more than I can handle.   *Mary*

I entered the room with tears just because of life's challenges, but the fact that God is on the throne, makes all things worthwhile.

So for now I sit and wait and wonder
On what the films will show.
I have no fear, I feel so calm,
For my savior, my boat shall row.

God is with you always. He will never leave you or forsake you. Be blessed.

Oh, to just trust in the Lord, regardless of the outcome.   *MA*

The test wasn't bad at all. I'm not even worried about the outcome. I have faith in God that everything will be alright. It is well with me.

Life is given by God. In him we should always trust. Today my trust is stronger than the day before, the week before, the month before, even the year before. Because today I found out I have cancer in my right breast. I am here again to have a left breast mammogram. My doctor wants to be sure nothing is forming in it. This word "cancer" is evil. It pulls your strength from you. It will shake your belief. But trust in God. He renews everything. To all the women who will walk through this door, always remember, there's hope. God bless. *AH*

And God said he would take care of us,
For us to ask and receive.
So, why all the fuss? *Christine R*

Remember no matter what the results of your exam, Allah is in charge of everything and he will supply all of your needs.

I had my first mammogram this year. I was scared at first but am not anymore. I just put my trust in God and he will see me through anything.

May God bless you and continue to get your mammograms. We women have so much to do when it comes to keeping our bodies healthy.

"By his stripes we are healed", Isaiah 53:5. Thank you for a few moments of pain and discomfort.

I am only twenty four years old and still a baby. Coming in for these multiple tests is kind of scary. Nevertheless, I know that Yahweh will take care of me. *Chevon*

Seriously, I am afraid of breast cancer and especially now at this point in my life. My hope does lie with my faith in God. I know he has plans for me. God bless, Ladies.

Early detection is what we want. A second set of diagnostics is good. The earlier an anomaly is found the stronger we can be.

The better the outcome is possible. God is with us through peaks, valleys, and cleavage! Think positive in all you do and choose to do for yourself!

Today the experience was much less painful than in the past. Thank God for new technology and machines. Took considerable less time also. An unpleasant experience in your life, could very well be life changing as in saving your life! God bless and have a happy healthy, life!   *BW*

```
Whatever the x-ray shows,
There's a God that always knows.
Why fret or be in fear,
When there's my Savior who's always near.
So, where is the lump?
Oh my dear, it was just a bump!      CN
```

Thank you, Lord, for this machine. Two lumps but no cancer. I pray for all who take advantage of this test.

God is wonderful, the mammogram was great! I came in with 2 breasts and left with 2 breasts!   *Brenda*

I had my yearly mammogram. Something was seen on it and the radiologist had to look at my films. Another film was taken.. As that second film was being read, I sat here and prayed. I prayed for the doctor reading the films. I asked God to let him know that I'm not just a number, but a child of the King. I prayed that God would use his hands and eyes as instruments from above so he would be God's tools. I sat and thought for a few minutes. God, is it my turn? Is my number up? My sister just finished radiation and my best friend has metastasized cancer throughout her body. Was it my turn today? I felt God's peace for whatever? The whatever was good news! Nothing! Let us all live each day to the fullest, by the grace of God! Praise God, my redeemer!   *Sue M*

Life is a gift from God. If he did not want man to help keep us healthy, He would not have allowed man to learn to build this machine. Isn't God wonderful?   *Carol D*

"Be patient under all conditions, and put your whole trust and confidence in God." Bahaullah   *a Baha'i friend*

GIRLS RULE!

Many patients are in the "sandwich generation". They're taking care of their parents, working, and have children in the home. They definitely have a full plate.

They're single, married, widowed, or divorced and doing their best to live a good life, pay bills, and taking care of all that life entails.

Starting their morning with us, dropping by during their lunch break, or after a long day is when many patients find the time to have a mammogram.

Frequently, coming in for a mammogram is their only "break" in the day, especially when they're caring for an elderly parent , ill spouse or relative. Unfortunately, taking care of themselves falls to the bottom of the list.

In spite of time restrictions, there's a lot of sharing that goes on between the patient and the mammographer. Women are natural bonders and connectors and the result is a feeling of sisterhood and understanding. We've laughed, we've cried, and our lives are made richer by each other.

If you really want to feel some sisterly power, join one of the walks offered against breast cancer. It is so awesome! It's a sea of women, babies, and men! You feel a big giant hug, lots of support, and even love! There may be t-shirts "In memory of", "In support of". There's survivors, families, friends together, all armed with hope and determination. Important information everywhere, healthy eats, souvenirs, and lots of joy and inspiration! Go! Walk! Run! Whatever! Do it for you, do it for loved ones, do it for women! Bring Kleenex, too! You will never forget the experience!

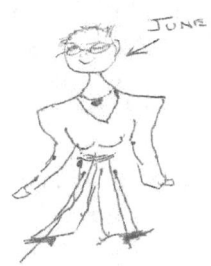

I'm thankful for my boobs that God gave me. This is getting easier each year! Keep the faith ladies, get the prettiest bras, and enjoy being a women! *Deb B*

Thank you! There is no possible way to ever complain about having this very simple procedure. Reading and realizing the struggle that these ladies and thousands more have everyday! They remain strong, so I certainly should too.

No doubt at forty seven years old, I'll be back. Remember, when life gives you lemons, for goodness sakes, make lemonade!
With love in friendship, *Janet*

Ah, the joys of womanhood!

I thank God for ladies like Elizabeth Edwards, who was able to share her experience with breast cancer to remind us that we should never fail to take care of ourselves.

Mammograms, just more evidence that we are the stronger sex.

Thank God for this big and powerful machine that has helped to save many a person's life! Even though, it may feel like a vice squishing me, it is a short-lived squash! I feel a part of the "Ya-Ya Sisterhood"! *Mary Helen*

We are blessed to have to do this only once a year. I can't wait for another invention, this time by a woman!

```
I had this done just once before.
Today, like then, I wanted to run for the
door.
But, "No", Doc says, "it's so
necessary".
She's had it done and seemed quite caring.
Upon her advice, referral in hand, I
got up the courage and came rolling in.
With a smile on my face, a prayer in my
heart,
a wonderful receptionist, and a technician
whom I heard was very, very, smart.
I made it through and said, "Thank you,
dear".
Made it on through past one more little
fear.
```

```
So mammos aren't the most pleasant of
necessities in each of our lives,
But thanks to those mammos, they've saved
many sisters, daughters, friends, and
wives.  MLF
```

I have gotten such a spiritual lift from reading all of those comments. We as women are such a wealth of wisdom, spirituality, humor, and love. Thank you one and all.

Women are like tea bags. You don't know their strength until you put them in hot water. With God's love and family/friends support, anything can be handled.

It's funny going through the routine and diagnostic mammograms, you feel so alone. But reading these notes, it makes you feel that you are a part of a sisterhood. Not alone at all. Women have come before you and others after! We are all connected. See you in six months. *Jan*

Good luck to all of you who find it's better to be safe than sorry. God bless. *AL*

Here's praying that for each of us that endure this machine, that it finds us healthy. For those who are lucky enough to have gone through this and it was found in time, it was a small price to pay for your life. Encourage all your friends to be tested. I know we can win this battle over breast cancer. Spread the word, early detection is the answer.

I'm 55 and retiring! What a good way to begin by celebrating, hopefully, good health. Know that each woman coming here, like I, faces the reality of the results of this test. Hopefully, all with graciousness, hope, faith, and joy of living each day fully!

Women, be brave, be strong. Just do it.

Why did Eve eat that apple? What we women have to go through, it's beyond the call of duty. Because of the pain we endure, it only makes us better than men. Amen.
I thank God for this machine and I am very lucky. But why isn't it called "Becky" instead of "Bucky"?!

Ladies, we owe it to ourselves and our families to have these tests. Bless all the women with breast cancer and a breakthrough will soon emerge!

These notes are wonderful! Only women facing life threatening news could still have a sense of humor as shared here. I'm a retake. Good news expected ! *BE*

Hope everyone passes this test!

```
I do believe that I am blessed
To have two fine and healthy breasts.
And though this test is not great joy,
I'm still awfully glad I'm not a boy!
```
Grace

Don't miss your annual appointments! Make time in your busy schedule to take care of yourself. *Catherine*

Thank you, ladies, for your comments. I will never again look at having a mammogram as something to dread, but something to be grateful for. *Betty*
I saw "YaYa Sisterhood" just last night with a group of friends. It's great to be a woman, even if we have to do these mammograms. *L Price*

At 55, it's great to be alive! And since I plan to see 65, and 75,
and even 85. I endure this few moments of discomfort. Take a
deep breath ladies, and live. God bless! *D Smith*

For all my sisters who pass through
with their thoughts the same as mine,
know that someone prays for you.
That this test will be your best,
and the pictures are "fine". *L*

The Lady in Pink.
I'm waiting here 'cause
there's a lump
and my doc said, "Don't wait".
The squeezing make me want to jump.
"Just do it," says my mate.
I'm not afraid of squeezing things
and lumps aren't always omens.
I'm grateful for the help it brings
and give thanks to Susan Komen!

Don't mind the pain.
I don't mind the strain.
I figure I have nothing to lose, but early
detection will help me gain!

Early detection is best in gaining victory!

Super Hero
The squishionator.
Able to bring women to tears
but moments later
erasing their fears.

A squish here, a squish there, then the news comes and we know whatever they say, we will work to fix it! Let's go!
Joanne C

No matter how different and unique every woman is, we all have this commonality, this reality, the blessings of our breasts. It's so easy to critique them and wish they were bigger or perkier or higher or whatever until something happens to make you feel that perhaps, the ones you have, the ones you've always wanted to change a little, this way or that way, may be in jeopardy. I now realize that my breasts are great! Not because they're big or plump or perky, but because they are mine, the ones God gave me. I am so thankful! I am glad to be a woman.

MAN AND THE MACHINE

When confronted by the mammogram compression at the yearly appointment, women's dislike for the machine is displaced to men.

But listen carefully, and I think you'll hear the humor and hopefully, the gratefulness for the machine that's trying to save our lives.

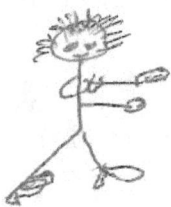

Not only was the machine designed by man, so was the bra! Someday we'll get even with man.

I don't know about you and how you feel about this machine. On one hand, I hate the machine, on the other hand every year, I look forward to the exam. It just doesn't seem fair that our husbands don't have to have a period, a baby, dye their hair, shave their legs, pluck their eyebrows, wear a bra or girdle, or have a mammogram! Boy, Eve really did us in didn't she?
Barbara

I hope one day, there is a machine for men so they can be rolled around, squeezed, and pulled apart!

I would love to see a man try to guess what a mammogram looks like in "Charades"!

Yes, let a man put his testicles into a vise. "Don't breathe", "Don't move". He would be singing soprano for weeks! And, yes, the machine had to be designed by a man.

We really need to find an equivalent of this test for men. They're missing so much of the joy that we have as women. Oh hell, we'll just nag them some more.

I know all the torment and torture we women have to go through is for our own benefit but collectively, we need to unite and slap the #### out of all the men who created these devices!

You know, men should have something squeezed in this machine, too, but I am not going to say what.   *Kay*

Men should be required to have yearly "manograms" or "ballograms" and put theirs in the machine. They would never return!
Pam

I wish men would have to do mammograms to see what women are going through. Especially, the male doctors who keep ordering this for us!

I have to have one of these mammograms every six months. They see something but they're not sure what. I told my husband, "It's so easy to be a man. No periods, no giving birth, no menopause, no mammograms, no birth control pills, no yearly pap smears and checkups, and no sagging boobs!" They have it made. I told him I wish just once he had to have his penis and balls squashed in a machine!!   *Dawn B*

I wish my husband could try this just once, even on his finger.

Thank God for the test but I think the contraption was designed by a man, just like three inch high heels and bras! Men have no idea what it's like to have a sensitive part smashed.

They can send a man to the moon, check the ocean floor with sonar but they have to mash my poor breasts to a pancake to get a good picture?! Priorities, huh? Seems that if a man had to do this annually, he'd think of something less painful. Oh well, good thing is that this one is ok and doesn't have breast cancer. Praise the Lord!

Ladies, this mammogram is about as much fun as your annual pelvic exam, which men also devised. P.S. It's really not that bad! It is better than breast cancer any day of the week.
K Nichols

There are many women I know with breast cancer. A little pain is tolerable to be told there is nothing wrong. Designed by a man, oh yes. Thanks. *Melissa*

SUGGESTION BOX

During the mammogram, I sometimes ask my patients whether they have any daughters or nieces. Hopefully by the time these young girls become old enough for mammograms, they'll have invented a "Star Trek" wand-like object, and these compressions will be a thing of the past!

So, if anyone has any ideas or suggestions for taking care of our breasts, pass it on! Chocolate might help.

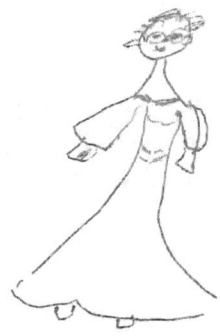

Why not set up a cappuccino bar so we can sip with our free hand while being smooshed by the machine?

I never dated anyone name"Bucky", let alone let him caress my breast.
Yet, I come here and we have a blind date.
He was a little heavy paddled, but I'm okay.

I hope next year they introduce me to a kinder, gentler, boob presser.
Can't say it's been great, "Bucky!"

I wish "Star War" technology would hurry up and get here before my next visit. *Karen*

```
Hey, look at it this way.
After all this squishing, you've surely lost
a calorie or two!
So go out and have a donut and caffeine brew!
```

I wonder who invented this "boob-squasher-machine"? There must be a better and more pleasant way to examine it, like a scanner. I think we should be treated with a full body massage. A little pampering to the babies, like good chocolates after this treatment! *Sarah*

If you ever clean your house in the nude and have been cooking in your oven, please, do not lean over to clean the top of the stove. Ouch!

I think it's time a woman invents a "bra-style-x-ray machine" that can deflate for bigger boobs or will inflate for smaller boobs. We could call it the "wonderbra mammogram"!
MaryBeth

I am grateful to be alive and very well. Maybe next time we'll have a new machine and one that doesn't need to press my booby!

How about a funny calendar of poses by willing participants?

This machine that man made feels like hell.
I hope someday that we'll invent something,
we'll design something,
that feels swell.

Glad this is only once a year. I'm looking for the day that we
don't have to be squished like pancakes.   *CS*

I think we should all bring our spouses or significant others.
I'm willing to bet they would be ever so tender with us always
and have some understanding of what it's like.

We need targeted exercise tips to get these things back up again!

Suggestions for improvements:
1.   Terrence Howard, shirtless, to take the mammo.
2.   Denzel Washington to kiss them and make them
     all better.
3.   Donald Trump to pay the bill!

AN INVITATION

I would love to hear from you. I'm sure you all have experiences, stories, and thoughts on having a mammogram that would be appreciated by others.

If you would like me to share them in another publishing, please send them to me and as soon as I gather enough responses I'll try to publish a volume 2!

Advise me how you want your name included and/or if you do not want your name or message published. Either way, I value your communications.

Please contact me at
www.tgionlyhave2ofthese.com.

Susan E Ghiassi R.T (R)(M)(CT) (ARRT)

NEWSFLASH!! DON'T MISS THIS!!!

IMPORTANT: Get a mammogram yearly beginning between the ages of 35-40. If possible, get a digital mammogram. If not, get what is available!

SPREAD THE WORD: If you get a letter saying come back for additional films, try not to panic. When you come back for additional films, we're really trying to see an area better that we weren't able to on the screening mammogram visit. By using different compression paddles or positioning, even ultrasound, aids the radiologist in reading your films. So stay calm and help us to take good films of your breast.

THE SIGNS OF BREAST CANCER MAY VARY AMONG WOMEN. Some breast cancers cannot be seen or felt. Check with your doctor if you have any of these symptoms:
> *lump, hard knot, or a thickening
> *change in breast size or shape
> *dimpling or puckering of the skin
> *itchy, scaly sore or rash on the nipple
> *a pulling in of the nipple or another part of the breast
> *nipple discharge that starts spontaneously
> *pain in one area you can point to with your finger
> *a swelling, warmness, redness, or darkening

A *"Free Mammogram Day"* is a great chance for an imaging facility to give back to the community. Raleigh Radiology Cedarhurst in Raleigh, NC has done this successfully for years during **October, Breast Cancer Awareness Month!**

The "Caring Community Foundation"
An organization that helps patients going through the cancer battle:
www.caringcommunityfoundation.org

See www.komen.org for breast health and breast cancer information

See www.sistersnetworkinc.org A national African-American breast cancer survivorship organization and a good source of information.

See www.helpfromhopp.org Butch Miller started Help from Hopp to aid cancer patients and honor his wife, who died of breast cancer. "to put a hand on a patient's shoulder to say someone cares".

YES, MEN CAN GET BREAST CANCER

It varies to how often we have a male patient come in for a mammogram. Diagnostic mammograms may be ordered for some of the same reasons female patients come in for an exam. Normally, when we have a male patient, we automatically do both sides for comparison.

The male patients are definitely uncomfortable, nervous and embarrassed. Sometimes it is a challenge to position the male breast, but the male patients are usually very cooperative and eager to know the results like the rest of us.

I always have one demand for my male patients. If you find this to be not painful at all or no big deal, do not leave this room thinking you can be unsympathetic to any female that feels differently. You still need to be compassionate. As one of my patients wrote, "My husband has had two mammograms. He understands."

INQUIRE WITHIN

Where you choose to have your mammogram is very important. Insurance coverage, the standard of care, and the radiologists that will be reading your films are all components that as a patient you need to investigate.

The dedicated mammography equipment, mammography records, and credentials are thoroughly inspected and strictly regulated by state and federal government offices. Through the Mammography Quality Standards Act (MQSA), a mammography site is required to maintain a Quality Assurance program that is inspected yearly by the Federal Drug Administration (FDA). Mammography facilities are accredited by the American College of Radiology (ACR).

Make sure the site where you plan to have your mammogram has passed the current inspections by the MQSA and has the ACR seal of approval.

In addition, if you are having a diagnostic mammogram it is necessary to have a radiologist on site to supervise the mammographer performing the exam.

LET'S GET TECHNICAL

A mammogram is a screening tool for breast cancer. The hope is the earlier you detect the breast cancer, the more treatable!

Between the ages of 35-40 you should get a baseline, screening mammogram. This is to have a set of films to compare to as a baseline for when you begin coming in for your yearly screening mammogram at 40 years old. The baseline (as well as the screening mammogram) generally consists of 2 views of each breast, totaling 4 films.

There are basically two types of mammograms: screening and diagnostic.

The screening or routine mammogram, normally done yearly, is the standard exam for the patient that is not having any problems with their breasts.

Before digital mammography, I would leave my patient to develop my screening mammogram films in the darkroom, saying, "I'm going to go check these to make sure I got good films before you leave. If I have to take some more, don't get alarmed. It doesn't mean I found anything, it just means I want to get a better picture." Now, with digital mammography, as a mammographer, you get to see and check the image almost instantly on the screen while still in the room with the patient.

After checking the films, patients know as mammographers, we can't give them results. The mammogram patient will receive a letter from the office indicating whether their results were alright or if they need to come back for additional views requiring a diagnostic mammogram. Their doctor usually gets a faxed report the same day with the report from the radiologist.

I always warn them that there's a chance they could get a letter saying come back for additional films. Don't get upset! It may be that the radiologist wants to see an area better or the film looks a little different from your previous ones. It happens more frequently when you're comparing older films with the new digital mammography films because of the difference in quality. Remember, most things are nothing.

The diagnostic mammogram is another story. The diagnostic mammogram is ordered because the radiologist has recommended additional films after reading the screening mammogram, or because the patient or their doctor has felt something new and different in the breast that needs further investigation. It could be because a family member, co-worker, or friend has recently received breast cancer news, and the patient becomes anxious about her own breasts. We know that the diagnostic mammogram patient is usually worried and scared.

For the diagnostic mammogram, the radiologist needs to be present in the office to read the diagnostic mammogram films.

For the patient coming back for additional films, the mammographer reads the radiologist's report which describes the films that need to be taken.

Upon completion of the diagnostic mammogram, we show our films to the radiologist. They may send us back to take some more or have us position the breast a little differently. Sometimes we need to change the equipment or the paddle, depending on the radiologist's requests. Ultrasound is another informational tool for the radiologist. They may even recommend that you come back in six months.

Sometimes the films are not definitive and the patient may need a biopsy.

After reviewing all the films, past and present, patient's history, and other information, the radiologist dictates his report. Some radiologists prefer to talk to the diagnostic patients. As mammographers we really appreciate the radiologist who speaks with our patients, as do the majority of patients. The waiting for the results plus the fear of the unknown is just awful.

There are also those patients that we feel would not be good candidates for receiving any news before leaving the office, and /or their doctor has notified our office that no results are to be given to their patients, so we act accordingly.

We realize it is just so hard to hear any news sometimes when you're blocked with apprehension and nervousness, so it's always better to have another set of ears to help you understand and ask questions.

We care. When it's bad news, we try to mask our feelings upon our return to the room, especially when the patient has to wait to speak with their doctor. We've held hands, patted shoulders, given hugs, and positive messages. Many times our eyes are filled with worry, or relief, depending on the results.

But listen, you've done everything you're supposed to do: You check your own breasts monthly, you have your doctor check your breasts yearly, and you get mammograms yearly. You helped me get good pictures

This is a very exciting time in medicine! The medicines are kinder and gentler. I've been told all this personally by a breast cancer researcher. He said in the near future we will have our DNA on a card and be able to go to the pharmacy and have medicine made just for us! It's happening!

The best times, of course, are when the radiologist tells the mammographer that we can tell the patient there are no problems, that they are fine! We're as glad as you are! The response is usually a cry of relief, tears of joy, with hugs and "thank you's".

It's important that you know I was able to get good quality mammogram films because you allowed me to move you around and compress your breast sufficiently. Thank you for your cooperation!

PREP TALK

As a patient there are steps you can take before your appointment that will help insure a successful mammogram.

It is important to do a breast self exam (BSE) monthly. Four to five days after your period has begun, or if you no longer have periods, just pick a date, and examine your breasts. You can pick up a "shower card" that reminds you and gives directions how best to check your breasts. You may be the one that detects something new in your breast!

Before your appointment, make sure you have seen your doctor or have discussed with them any problems you have with your breasts so that the appropriate exam is ordered.

Sometimes it's difficult to know what you are feeling in your breast, so here's a suggestion I got from one of my patients. When you visit your doctor, draw a sketch of your breasts like the one you find on the history sheet you fill out for your mammogram. Have the doctor spend time with you and ask questions. Mark the sketch of your breasts with the help of your doctor as to where the moles, cysts, and previous surgery scars are located. Also, feel your breasts and ask questions about what is normal to feel in a breast. When you're home alone, you'll have something to refer back to as to what was felt by the doctor and yourself. This may be helpful in case you feel something new in your breast.

To possibly avoid having unnecessary films done, know where your previous films are located and have them sent to the site before your appointment or have them in hand for the mammogram appointment. It's best to have your films all in one place so that the radiologist can compare your previous films with your present films for any changes in your breast.

It is recommended if you still menstruate, make your appointment 4 to 5 days after your period has begun, or if you no longer menstruate, just pick a date. Schedule it for when your breasts aren't so tender that you can't take any compression. If your breasts become tender from too much caffeine, cut down or eliminate it before your mammogram appointment.

Check with your insurance company to make sure you understand their policy for mammograms before you schedule your appointment.

When you make your mammogram appointment, you need to let the scheduler know if you have breast implants because it does require more time and films, 8 films instead of 4 films. Also, if you're unable to stand for too long, or if you're in a wheelchair, it's best to let the scheduler know and that way they can set more time aside for your exam.

If you have any open sores or cuts on your breast, and you're scheduled for a screening mammogram, maybe it would be better to schedule it for another day.

If you're still nursing your baby, and you're not having any problems with your breasts, it's better if you wait six months after you've stopped nursing to make an mammogram appointment.

On the day of your appointment wear a two piece outfit, it just makes it easier on you and allows you to be more covered up during the exam.

Do not wear any deodorant, powder, or sparkly lotion on your breast area for the exam. The reason for this is that ingredients in the deodorant or lotion may be mistaken for something more serious on the film.

Show the mammographer any large moles, scars, or previous surgeries on your breast. Point out the area that you or your doctor feels a lump. If you have breast implants, make sure you tell the mammographer.

It's important that you understand during a mammogram, the more you compress the breast with the paddle, the better the films and the less radiation the patient receives.

If you're up on your toes, or something is really pinching or poking you during the exam, don't hesitate to let the mammographer know. Maybe they can move you a little and are unaware of the problem.

Expect some pressure or discomfort, but it shouldn't be unbearable. Thank goodness you're not compressed for long, and it's an automatic release after the image is taken!! It does go quickly.

We need to work together to get the best films.

Knowing your own breasts by monthly self breast exams, having your yearly breast exam with your doctor, and having a mammogram every year from 40 years of age, altogether is your best insurance for early detection. Neither one alone is enough.

GLOSSARY

*FOR A VALUABLE SOURCE OF CURRENT INFORMATION ON BREAST HEALTH AND BREAST CANCER, GO TO : www.komen.org

Baseline mammogram- between 35-40 years old is when a woman generally has her first mammogram done. It is used for comparison to the future yearly mammograms.

Benign-Not cancer; Not malignant

Biopsy- surgical removal and microscopic examination of tissue to see if cancer cells are present.

Black women and breast cancer- White women usually have the highest rates of breast cancer, followed by African-Americans, Asian-Americans/Pacific Islanders, Hispanics/Latinas and American Indians/Alaskan Natives. White women are more likely to develop post-menopausal breast cancer. African-American women are more likely to develop pre-menopausal breast cancer. ***For African-Americans, a wonderful source of information and support for breast cancer is the** www.sistersnetworkinc.org.

Breast lift-removes excess skin and reshapes remaining tissues.

Bucky-the breast is placed upon the bucky. It is the imaging area. Sometimes holds the cassettes.

CAD (computer aided detection)-computer based tool that assists radiologists in the interpretation of mammograms.

Caffeine effects-caffeine may cause breast to be more tender. Caffeine is found in tea, coffee, soda, chocolate, to name a few.

Cancer-abnormal growth of cells; divide without control and are able to invade other tissues. Malignant.

Caring Community Foundation-an organization that began with a "paying it forward" idea to help someone who has been diagnosed with breast cancer. ***For more information:** www.info.caringcommunityfoundation.org.

Charades-a fun game where people try to guess the movie, book, person, etc., by clues given by pantomime and a specific sign language. No mouthing of words or talking is allowed.

Chemo (Chemotherapy)-Drugs that destroy or slow down the growth of the cancer cells. Sometimes they are used before the surgery, and sometimes afterwards. They can be taken orally as tablets or capsules, but usually, they're injected into a vein.

Cyst-Fluid filled sacs that are almost always benign. Sometimes a patient can feel them. They can be seen on the mammogram and with ultrasound.

Diagnostic mammogram-a patient's doctor may have felt an area that needs further investigation, the patient has felt something, or an abnormal finding from a screening mammogram has been found by a radiologist and the patient will need additional films. The radiologist needs to be on site to supervise the mammographer taking the films for a diagnostic mammogram.

Diagram- refers to the diagram guidelines seen on the compression paddle.

Dolly Parton- beloved buxom country singer!

Elizabeth Edwards- wife of former senator from North Carolina, John Edwards, who went public with her diagnosis of breast cancer. **Note: Robin Roberts** and **Hoda Kotb** of the morning news shows, **Melissa Ethridge** and **Sheryl Crow**, singers, etc., are a few of the woman in the public eye who have also gone public with their breast cancer diagnosis. **Kay Yow**, beloved basketball coach for NCState, went public and her foundation helps raise money for the battle against breast cancer. This definitely has a positive effect on women to come in for mammograms as well as to be hopeful and positive for their own futures. I think it's great!

Eve-from the biblical story in Genesis

Howard, Terrence-actor

In situ (DCIS)-also known as intraductal non-invasive breast disease or stage 0 breast cancer. It is a pre-cancerous condition. The abnormal cells remain inside the lobules or milk ducts.

Komen, Susan-Nancy G Brinker promised her older sister, Susan G Komen, that she would do everything in her power to end breast cancer forever.

Lymphedema-fluid collects in the arm, causing swelling, caused by the removal of axillary lymph nodes or radiation therapy.

Lumpectomy-also referred to as breast conserving surgery or wide excision. Generally, the patient has had a cancerous mass removed. Minimal breast tissue is removed.

Male breast cancer-men can also develop breast cancer, though it is much rarer. For men, the tumor is most often under the nipple and the main treatment is mastectomy. 1 in 1,000 for men while 1 in 8 for women.

Malignant- a malignant tumor is cancer; description of cancer.

Mammogram-technique using x-rays to provide image of the breast. Tumors, microcalcifications, and abnormal skin changes can be seen. Best screening tool for breast cancer.

Mammogram before age 40-may be necessary if patient has: **1.** mutation (changes) in the genes called, **BRCA1** or **BRCA2** (short for breast cancer 1 and breast cancer 2). **2.** Very strong family history such as mother and/or sister diagnosis at age 40 or less. **3.** Personal history of breast cancer, atypical hyperplasia, radiation treatment on chest area during childhood or young adulthood.

Metastasis-spread of cancer from one part of the body to another. Metastasize means if a cancer spread.

Modified radical mastectomy-surgeon removes one breast, lining of the chest muscles and some lymph nodes in the armpit (called axillary dissection). This type is used to treat invasive cancers, including early breast cancer, locally advanced breast cancer, inflammatory breast cancer, and Paget's disease with underlying invasive disease.

MRI (magnetic resonance imaging)-uses magnetic field to create an image of the breast. Contrast agent is injected to help with diagnosis. Higher risk women due to **BRCA1** or **BRCA2**, or strong family history, benefit from MRI.

"No one in my family"-85% of breast cancers found are in women with **no** family history.

Poem-"Ode to Mammogram", author anonymous.

Power failure-during a mammogram a separate override feature will automatically relieve the compression.

Radiation-radiation therapy is often used to destroy any remaining breast cancer cells in the breast, chest wall, or axilla (underarm) after surgery. Treatment using high energy rays to damage (burn) cancer cells and stop them from growing.

RRC (Raleigh Radiology Cedarhurst)-a full service, outpatient radiology facility in Raleigh, North Carolina

Reconstruction-breast reconstruction can help restore the look and feel of the breast after mastectomy, done by a plastic surgeon. There are 2 types: one uses artificial implants and one uses skin and tissue from the woman's own body.

Retake (additional films, diagnostic films)-are ordered as a diagnostic unilateral(one side) or bilateral(both sides) mammogram. The radiologist has made a decision to follow-up with more mammogram films in order to see some area(s) better and it may be followed by an ultrasound.

Screening mammogram (routine or yearly mammogram)-beginning at 35-40 years of age and continuing every year, and when a patient is not having any problems with her breasts detects early signs of breast cancer.

BSE (breast self exam)-once a month, 4-5 days after the start of menstruation, a woman should check her own breast by looking in the mirror to see any changes and by a combination of pressing and moving the hand over the entire breast area and beyond to feel for any breast changes.

Shower card- a plastic card that you can hang in the shower that demonstrates how to do a breast self exam.

Six month follow-up- is one recommendation made by the radiologist. The patient would return in six months for more films to check the area of concern.

Sonogram (ultrasound)– diagnostic test that uses sound waves to create images of tissues and organs. Tissues of different densities reflect sound waves differently. Breast ultrasonography is best utilized for cystic versus solid differentiation. It can distinguish a liquid filled cyst from a solid mass. It helps to distinguish the difference between normal and abnormal breast lumps. Commonly used in addition to the diagnostic mammogram.

Stage 1-doctors use rating scale to describe breast cancer. The higher the stage or number, the more extensive the cancer. The scale includes 0,l,ll,lll, and lV. The scale is dependent on the size of the tumor, whether the cancer has spread to the axilliary nodes (glands in the underarm), and signs of metastasis (cancer spreading to other parts of the body). It helps determine appropriate treatment options.

Star Trek- TV series about exploring new worlds in space.

Susan G Komen for the Cure- an organization fighting to cure breast cancer since 1982. More information can be found at www.komen.org.

Trump, Donald- American business tycoon.

Total mastectomy (simple mastectomy)-surgeon removes entire breast but no other tissue or node. Used for treatment of ductal carcinoma in situ, Pagets disease with underlying non-invasive cancer and in some cases, recurrent breast cancer.

Tumor- mass of extra tissue. Can be cancerous (malignant) or benign (no cancer).

Washington, Denzel- actor

Wonderbra- brand of bra

Ya Ya Sisterhood- a story about 4 ladies and their friendship and alliance through the years.

Yahweh = God, Lord, Allah

A LITTLE HISTORY

Discover for your self, there have been many more surgeons, radiologists, scientists, and inventors than are noted below that have played a part in the creation of the mammogram! The quest continues today with more research, testing, and debating.

1895   William Roentgen, a German physicist, discovers x-rays
1913   Albert Solomon, a German surgeon, uses a conventional x-ray machine to   visualize breast cancers in 3000 mastectomy specimens.
1940   Stafford Warren, a radiologist in New York, develops a stereoscopic system for tumor identification
1949   Raul Leborgne, a Uruguayan, emphasizes the need for breast compression to identify calcifications. Charles Gros, a radiologist in Strasbourg, France, develops the first radiological unit designed to examine breasts.
1957   Robert Egan, a radiologist in Houston, introduces dedicated film for mammography which improves detail. Also, he determines there's a need for trained mammogram technicians and radiologists to produce the quality film and accurate readings.
1966   First dedicated mammography machine is developed
1970's- Several manufacturers begin selling dedicated mammography systems: Siemens, Philips, Picker
1980's-1990's Major advancements in mammography equipment such as reduced radiation dosage, better film, digital imaging, and computer-aided detection.
Digital spot view mammography is developed to allow faster and more accurate stereotactic biopsies than traditional biopsies.

2000   First full field digital mammography system is introduced

2001   Study of digital mammography versus standard film mammography

Presently, (2009), digital mammography is recommended.

CITATIONS

www.komen.org was a source of information African-American women breast cancer, male breast cancer, and some of the definitions in the glossary.

Sarah Kenefick R.T.(R)(M) (ARRT), Diagnostic Team Leader at Raleigh Radiology Cedarhurst, Raleigh, North Carolina.

Susan E. Ghiassi (nee Miller) was born in St. Louis, Missouri, graduated from the Radiologic Technology Career Program at SLCC-Forest Park in 1980. Worked as a radiological technologist/mammographer/CT technologist at Deaconess Hospital, and Central CT & Radiology in St. Louis. In Raleigh, North Carolina, since 1996, worked as a mammographer/radiological technologist at Kaiser Permanente and is presently employed as a mammographer/radiological technologist at Raleigh Radiology Cedarhurst and Duke Raleigh Hospital. She resides in Raleigh, North Carolina, with her husband, Rasool, enjoying visits and stories from their sons, Ali and Hassan, as they begin their own lives.